DIY 101 Yummy

Organic e-Juice

Recipes

By

Roland Harrison

Published by:

www.Valenciapub.com

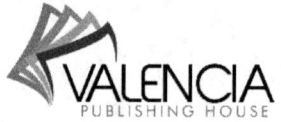

Valencia Publishing House

P.O. Box 548

Wilmer, Alabama 36587

Cover & Interior designed

By

Alex Lockridge

First Edition

What's In This Book?

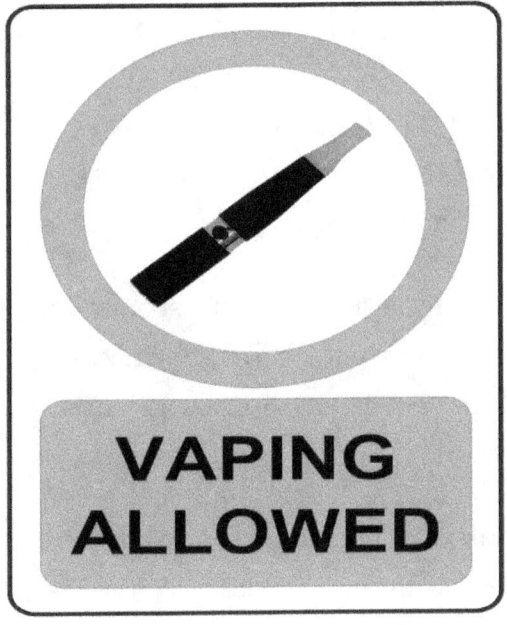

Foreword

LATELY, my new found obsession is everything Organic, especially vaping organic e-juice. I am an avid vaper and have been vaping, selling, importing, retailing, wholesaling e- cigarettes for last six years now. But this is not about my success or failure in business; it is about vaping the yummy e-liquids.

Let me ask, have you tried any organic e-juice yet? Well if you haven't, you are missing out and I think you owe it to yourself to at least make a few flavors yourself and try them.

You may ask why I should make my own when I can just order from an online retailer right? In case you haven't noticed, the prices of e-liquids have doubled in last two years, especially if you are buying the US made organic e-juice.

Last time I bought a 30ml bottle of an organic e-juice I paid $27.50 plus shipping!! I have been making my own eojuice for four years now, and I suggest you try making a batch too. Trust me it can be an awesome and fun experience to be able to create something you can call your own brand. But more importantly, the cost savings can be reason enough that you would want to start making your own.

Just to give you an example, to make a 30ml bottle of any flavor of organic e-juice at home can cost you around $3-$5 depending on what flavoring you use. Now to buy same the quality and quantity e-juice from any reputable online or local retailers can cost you $20-$28. The difference is $23!!!!!!!!!!

When you vape store bought liquid, do you ever say, "I wish they added one more drop of menthol or little more coffee flavor to this juice"? Well when you make your own, you don't have to wish that anymore, just add more or be more creative and mix a few recipes together and come up with a unique one that has your signature on it.

If you end up making a few great recipes, you can even start your own brand and try to market them as premium organic e-juice online and have a business that you never thought you would have. The possibilities are endless!

Preparing your perfect e-juice recipe and getting all the ingredients in the right quantity is quite a bit of work. It requires patience and constant trial and error to reach the goal, and until you're done perfecting one recipe, you may be exhausted, and unwilling try further. Experimenting with making your own e-juice can thus, result in a tenuous experiment that drains your energy in the end and leaves you shoving it aside, only to find yourself saving and spending money on pre-made e-liquid that you are bound to buy.

But wait, things don't have to be that bad, and you don't have to exhaust yourself trying to perfect your e-liquid recipes. I have gone through the trouble for you because I was keen to learn and perfect my art of e-juice for myself and my friends, and I'm ready to share it here with you!

After spending hours, days, and months I have perfected some great tasting super yummy e-juice recipes that you all will love to try as well. I am sure of it because my friends already can't get enough of them.

Whether or not you are an avid e-cigarette smoker, this book right here is for you!

What does this book include?

This book covers the basics of preparing e-juices by yourself as well as the ingredients that are required in detail, as those who are new to it can find it difficult to adjust to the terms and ingredients as they are a bit different from conventional cigarette ingredients.

Once you understand the basics of the ingredients, we will cover the equipment required, which isn't much. It is easy, and you can do it with a bit of effort.

Next up, once you are ready, you can get started with the recipes where I bring tried and tested e-liquid recipes to you that are sure to elevate your vaping experience to a whole new level. There isn't one or two, but five different categories of organic e-juice recipe flavors that I have covered in this book. You will find it interesting to explore recipes in the following flavor categories:

- Real Fruit Flavored Recipes
- Bakery Flavored Recipes
- Yummy Dessert Flavored Recipes
- Sweet Candy Flavored Recipes

- Truly Awesome Drink Flavored Recipes

Now I'm sure you're excited to get your hands on your e-juice in these exciting recipe flavor categories, so without further ado, let's get started. Shall we?

Introduction

THE VAPING community is full of choices and tastes, but it is also about personalization and individuality. Whether you are new to vaping or have been doing it awhile; you'll eventually think of a flavor you want, but can't find. Finding a vape that you enjoy is difficult enough, but finding one that is exactly what you want is near to impossible. That is why you need to consider making your own organic e-juice.

Making your own e-juice is similar to making cookies. You will need ingredients, some basic equipment and some instructions and recipes to put everything together. From this basic area, you can experiment as much as you want until you get the e-juice you love that is all your own.

Vaping is as much about great taste choices as it is about individuality and I understand that, as with everything else in life that quickly loses its charm, your once favorite eJuices may have too!

We're getting to the recipes but before we nose dive into them, let me touch upon the main ingredients and the equipment you will need to prepare your recipe. I want you to understand that perfecting and crafting a new flavor of eJuices is an art, and that takes time. Understanding what a recipe is made of will better equip you with the knowledge and understanding of the recipe itself.

With practice, you may even start to understand how you can alter the ingredients' ratio to create a mild or stronger flavor and all that will come when you understand the dynamics of the underlying ingredients

E-Juice Ingredients You Need

Diluted Nicotine

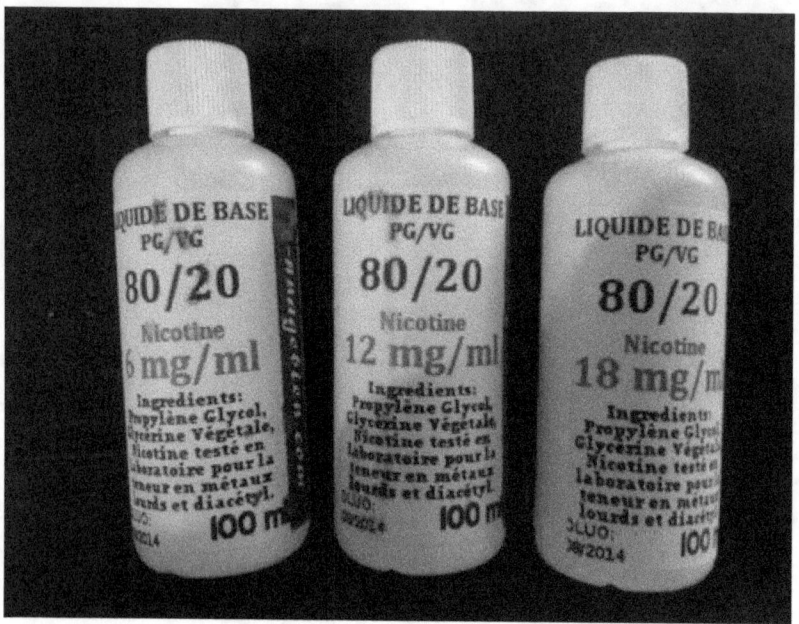

NICOTINE HAS a flavor to itself, so your recipes will taste different based on the strength of the nicotine. Generally, the e-juice industry uses 100mg/ml diluted nicotine because it makes it easier to calculate a specific strength per volume. Also, a small amount of 100mg/ml will go a long way and provide your more flexibility in your diluent ratio. Pure nicotine is 1000mg/ml and requires special equipment to handle including a specialized hazmat suit and a ventilation hood. Nicotine is dangerous at high concentrations both through skin contact and inhalation. If you aren't sure about mathematics or ability to handle safely, then you should stick with 25mg/ml nicotine. We'll discuss how you can make your own nicotine juice from tobacco leaf later, but it is important that when working with nicotine you take all precautionary measures.

PG or VG

In addition to nicotine, you are going to need either propylene glycol or vegetable glycerin as a diluent. Both nicotine and flavorings are highly concentrated and need to be diluted to have a good vaping experience. When making up your formula, the majority of the volume will be PG or VG as the base or carrier fluid.

There are a few slight differences between PG and VG. They both have slightly different tastes, viscosities and throat feel when vaped. Most e-liquids you purchase on the market have a mix of both and is represented as a ratio of PG to VG. Common ratios are 70/30, 50/50 or 30/70. Flavor concentrates are often diluted with PG. Both PG and VG are fine for vaping, but you'll probably want to use a little bit of both and experience with different ratios when you first get started with making your own e-juice.

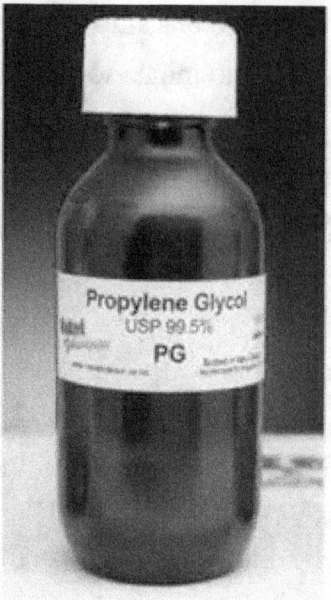

PG is an organic chemical compound that is often used in food, tobacco, and personal care products. It is also used in topical, oral, injectable and inhaled medications. PG won't alter the true flavor of flavor concentrates as much as VG. PG also offers a stronger throat hit, which can cause a slight irritation after extended use. Although rare, some people have developed allergies to PG.

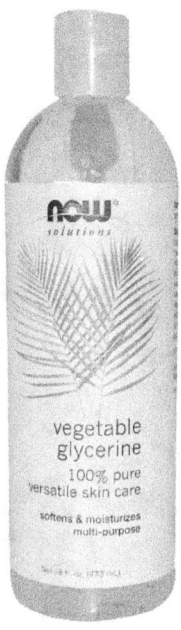

VG is slightly sweeter and more viscous or thicker than PG. VG can slightly alter the flavor either good or bad depending on individual tastes. High VG is usually preferred by those using cotton and coil atomizers since it has a smoother throat feel and generates a more visible cloud.

Flavors

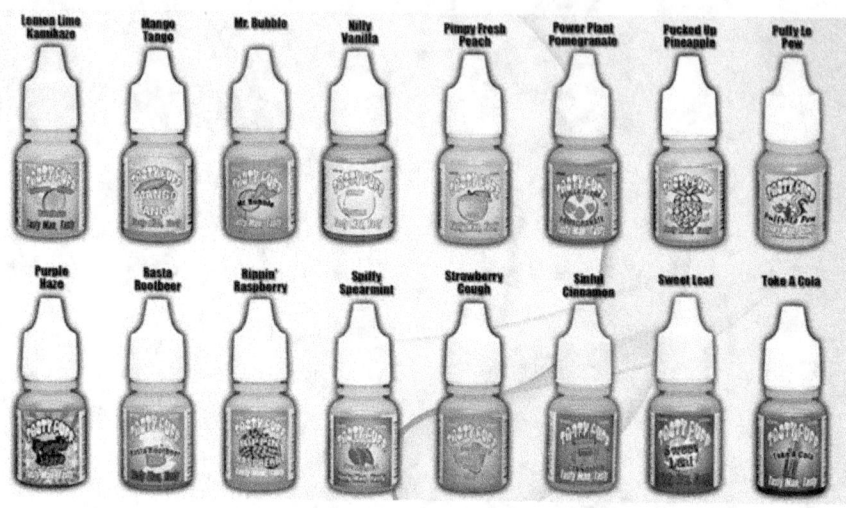

(Image is from HerbalVapeShop.com)

The last thing you need is, of course, flavors. You can get flavors from a variety of sources when creating a unique formula. In addition, to a wide range of flavors you can choose from, there is also the option of making e-juice without flavor. This is known as neat e-liquid. This isn't a common vape choice, but you can try it to see if is for you. But remember it is the flavors that makes the ultimate difference. Also, this is the ingredient that makes a juice organic as long as you buy the true organic flavor extract liquid. I will explain more on this in next chapter.

Color

One important thing to remember about color of your juice is, try your best to have no color at all, what I mean by that is the clearer the liquid is the longer your atomizers will last and vice versa. Dark color clogs atomizers faster. Now you may wonder, when you buy a banana flavor liquid from your local shop why it looks yellowish but when you make it, it looks pale or at least not yellow. Well, because they add color to the liquid to make it look more appealing to the eye. But you don't have to do that, keep it as natural as you can. This way you will vape one fewer chemical.

What Will Make your e-Juice Organic?

FIRST, AS you understand there are three main ingredients that go into each e-juice recipe, and they are a VG/pg blend, liquid nicotine juice, and flavor extracts, right?

VG is Vegetable Glycerin, USDA food grade VG is the best one to buy, but is it organic? No, not really, but don't get mad at me, wait let me finish. Let's talk about PG now which is propylene glycol; this is a harmless consumable chemical and as we all know chemicals can't be organic right? Just remember that both PG and VG are considered non-toxic, and FDA says they are "Generally Recognized as Safe."

Now, as for the nicotine juice, unless you want to soak a tobacco leaf and extract juice that way, the one you buy from the online stores are typically diluted as I mentioned above, and it is usually just diluted with either VG or PG or even with a blend of the both.

But what makes an e-liquid organic is a flavor extracts that you add what makes it organic. If you use organic fruit extract for flavoring, then the juice will be organic e-juice.

Now there are ways you can make the flavor extracts at home, but it is a long and tedious process, and you will need some technical know how to do that. Instead what we do is we find a good reputable retailer that sells these organic flavor extracts and simple use those when we make our organic e-juice.

Anytime you see an ad for organic e-juice, that is what it is. But remember those organic flavorings can be on the pricey side, but the good thing is you don't have to use a lot of them, so one 15-20ml bottle will be able to last you a few 50ml e-juice bottles, as you only have to add just a few drops of each flavor in each bottle.

E-Juice Equipment

Bottles

A T A MINIMUM, you are going to need some bottles. Plastic drip tip bottles are the most cost effective option when you are experimenting with e-juice recipes. This is because getting bottles clean enough to re-use for different flavors is often more work than it is worth. However, when you have a smaller bottle, you need to make sure your math and measurements are precise. It may be harder to measure small quantities accurately.

Containers

If you move on to making larger quantities, then you'll want to get some graduated cylinders or beakers. These are great for preventing cross contamination if you have a limited number of syringes.

Syringes

Both syringes and pipettes are an important tool for helping you with small openings on containers and getting the right amount of liquid from your supply into your e-juice creation. They allow you to extract exactly the right amount of nicotine, PG/VG or flavor you need and transfer it to a mixing container.

Gloves

Nicotine can be absorbed through the skin and spills are going to happen occasionally, therefore it is important to have gloves while you're working.

If you watch the YouTube video I mention in the next chapter, you will get to see every one of these items in action.

How to Make Pure Nicotine

I T IS POSSIBLE to make your own nicotine from tobacco leaves. However, I would caution against doing this since nicotine in its pure form is one of the deadliest poisons. Pure nicotine should not be ingested and can be absorbed through the skin, so you need to protect yourself if you are going to strain pure nicotine from plants. Let's look at this easy but dangerous process.

You need to start with tobacco leaves, or you can use chewing or pipe tobacco. All of these contain nicotine.

Place the tobacco in a bowl and fill with just enough water to cover and let it soak overnight.

Strain the mixture through a paper towel into a pot. After all of the slurries has been poured out, wring out the paper towel into the pot. Avoid letting any of the grounds or leaves fall out of the paper towel. Throw away the paper towel and leaves or grounds.

Now boil the liquid. The more water that boils away, the purer the nicotine.

Collect the nicotine with a spoon or scraper. Store in a sealable container. The nicotine should be the consistency of syrup and needs to be handled with caution. It is recommended you wear both eye and hand protection at least or a full hazmat suit at best.

Here is a video on YouTube where a guy shows how he made nicotine juice from a cigar, take a look. He actually makes a cigar flavor e-juice at the end.

https://www.youtube.com/watch?v=nRH9bBU0YMg

The Process of Making E-Juice

N O MATTER what recipe you choose to try you are going to follow a specific process to make your e-juice. You won't get the ideal flavor on your first try. It can take several tries to get it right. Take careful notes and precise measurements are you work so you can reproduce it later or know what you've tried before. The following is the step-by-step process for making e-juice.

Step 1: Nicotine Strength

The first step you need to take is to determine the strength of the nicotine you want in your e-juice, then figure out how much nicotine you need. The math isn't that difficult, but if you get it wrong, it could cause an unpleasant experience.

First, you want to determine how many milligrams of nicotine you need:

(Strength in mg/ml) (Volume in ml) = Amount of nicotine in mg

For example:

You want to make 50 ml of 8mg/ml e-juice.

So you need 50x8=400mgs of nicotine for a 50 ml formula.

Next, you need to determine the volume you need to use:

(Amount needed) / (Strength of diluted nicotine) = Volume to use

For example:

You have 100mg/ml diluted nicotine

So you need 400mg / (100mg/ml) = 4ml

You have 25mg/ml diluted nicotine

So you need 400 mg / (25mg/ml) = 16ml

Here is a YouTube video where a guy shows how he makes his e-juice. It is a helpful video, do take a look at it.

https://www.youtube.com/watch?v=YhCsugDc74c

Step 2: Extracting Nicotine

For this step, you need to put on gloves and transfer the nicotine to your bottle. You need to make 8mg/ml, and you have 25mg/ml PG nicotine. You have a 50ml bottle. Using a clean syringe, you should extract 16ml from your nicotine container.

Drawing the right amount can be difficult, so the easiest way is to pull the plunger back until you have a little more than needed then carefully depress back to the 16ml mark. Keep the syringe pointed into the container of nicotine when depressing so you can prevent wasting any diluted nicotine.

Air bubbles in the syringe can throw off measurements. If there is any air in the syringe, point the needle up and tap the syringe to move the air to the top then carefully depress the plunger until the liquid just starts to appear at the needle tip. Then you can point the needle back into the container and depress the plunger until you get to the right measurement.

Step 3: Transfer Nicotine

Once you have the amount you need in the syringe, simply squirt the nicotine into your 50ml bottle.

Step 4: Choose Your Flavors

You can choose any flavor combination you want or follow one of the combinations in the recipes later in this book.

Step 5: Measure and Transfer the Flavor

The recommended dilution for e-flavors is 10%, so if you're making 50 ml, you would need 5ml. Use a different and clean syringe for measuring and transferring the flavor concentrate to the bottle just like you did for the nicotine.

Be aware that flavor concentrates are tricky. Adding more flavor isn't going to make it better. Over flavoring e-juice can wash out the flavor and make it taste more like chemical constituents rather than the flavor you were going for. When using e-flavors, it is best to keep the total volume of all the flavors at 10-15% of the total volume of e-juice.

It is also important to note that when you mix multiple flavors, they can come out tasting different than what you'd expect; either good or bad. Sometimes you only need a hint of a flavor in order to bring out or balance the other flavors. As you experiment, you will notice this effect. Sometimes you may want to try a flavor by itself with just PG/VG base to get a sense of the flavor before adding it to a recipe.

Step 6: Measure and Add the Diluent/Base

To complete your liquid, you need to add the diluent/base. The e-juice is already going to have a lot of PG from the nicotine and flavoring so you are best using VG.

From our example above: we've added 16 ml of diluted nicotine and 5mls of flavoring for a total of 21mls. You still need 29mls to match calculations for 50mls total. Use a different and clean syringe to transfer 29mls of VG to your bottle.

It is important to note that bottles aren't graduated or don't have measuring marks. They tend to hold slightly more than the volume they are labeled with. Bottles can also vary in shape and total volume depending on the manufacturer. If you have several bottles, you can fill one with 50mls of water to see how full it should be when you are doing making your e-juice.

If you want a specific PG/VG blend ratio, you can do some quick math to determine how much of each to add. For 50/50 you would need 4mls more PG and 25mls of VG. To make a higher VG blend than the 42/58 we created you could use a higher strength of diluted nicotine to reduce the total amount of PG or you can use nicotine diluted with VG.

Step 7: Cap The bottle and Shake

Now you want to shake the bottle for several minutes to evenly disperse the nicotine and flavor. You should also shake it before each vape since the components can separate over time.

Step 8: Steep, Wait and Use

Your e-juice is now basically ready to vape, but the flavor may not be exactly what you were expecting. If you've ever cooked anything with seasonings, you know that the flavors really start to come out and change dramatically after a day or two in refrigeration or a few hours of slow cooking.

With e-juice, this is known as steeping. Steeping allows the chemical reactions to take place between the ingredients and oxygen. This allows the flavors to blend. A little time will make a big difference in flavor. Most e-juices need to steep for at least a few days and possibly even weeks. Once you shake it, take the cap off and let it sit for a few days. This is particularly important when working with flavors such as creams, vanillas, custards or fruits.

The Perfect Blend

BEFORE WE start talking about recipes, one important point I want to make is about the perfect blend of VG/PG. The truth is there is none. Depending on your personal preference and the type of atomizers you use, you may like 50-50 ratio like I do in some juice and in others, I like 60-40 where 60% VG and 40% PG. Just remember if you use atomizers that don't like thicker heavier juice then reduce your VG and increase PG. PG is lighter and more water like than VG.

Now as for the difference in vaping, PG will give you more throat hit while VG will produce a white cloud like smokes. If you are a smoker who used to smoke Marlboro lights, then you want a nicotine strength of 12mg to 18mg but never higher. If you smoke full flavor cigarettes then you want to try 18-24mg and if you an ultra-light cigarette smoker than try 6-12mg.

My Advice

Okay, next, you must be wondering where you are going to get all these supplies from right? Well, there are hundreds of online and local retail shops that sell all the ingredients. You can source some locally, some online.

But here is my advice. You should always buy USDA food grade VG, USP grade PG only. As for nicotine juice, it is up to you; you can make your own or buy ones already made, when buying nicotine juice, make sure to buy from a reputable vendor, this way you know you will be getting the real stuff. Always use a calculator and a precise measuring syringe to figure out the exact measurement of all liquids.

For example, if the recipe calls for 5% of some flavor, what is that 5% translate to in terms of liquid? How much is 5%? Well, it depends on how much total volume you are making. Say you are making 50ml of some liquid okay? So 5% of 50 ml should be 2.5 ml. You should have a syringe that can measure this 2.5 ml precisely, as little variations in flavorings can make a huge difference in taste.

Another advice is, if you are just starting out, don't try to make a recipe that calls for more than two flavorings, start out with a few simple ones that you think you may like first, and see how the process works. Once you are comfortable, then go all out experiment till your heart is content. But start out easy and simple this way you will stay motivated. Remember it is not only for fun, but to save money too.

All the supplies you need (gloves, syringes, etc.) you can pick them up locally or order online, they will not make any difference. But what will make the difference is where you buy your flavors from.

That is what makes or breaks e-juice quality. It is not the VG, nor the PG it is always the flavorings that make the juice great. So do your research and see who offers the flavors you like and has a good reputation for it.

At the end of this book I will mention a couple of names I bought from, but since there are so many online retailers, I don't want to give any of them an unnecessary boost and free advertising. Because my fear is, once I mention their names, and people start buying from them what if their quality goes down the drain? I will bear some of that blame for sure because I recommended them right?

Now let's go make some juice...

E-Juice Recipes

Fruit Flavors

All About Melons

Start with PG/VG/Nicotine base of your choice and add:

- ➤ Cantaloupe 5%

- ➤ Sweet Watermelon 5%

- ➤ Honeydew 5%

- ➤ Cream or Vanilla 5%

- ➤ Ethyl Maltol (10% mixture in 100% VG) 10%

- ➤ Sweetener 5%

Steep 48 hours.

Creamy Dragon/Pear

Start with PG/VG/Nicotine base of your choice and add:

- ➤ Pear 5%

- ➤ Cream 5%

- ➤ Dragon Fruit 5%

Shake for about 45 seconds and a quick hot bath. Wait 15 minutes.

Sweet Punch

Start with PG/VG/Nicotine based on your choice and add:

➢ Orange 5%

➢ Lemon Lime 5%

➢ Watermelon 2%

➢ Cranberry 2%

➢ Coconut Candy 1%

Let steep for a few days.

Fruit Custard

Start with PG/VG/Nicotine based on your choice and add:

➢ Dragon Fruit 5%

➢ Watermelon 10%

➢ Vanilla Custard 2%

Steep 7-14 days.

Creamy Orange/Pineapple

Start with PG/VG/Nicotine based on your choice and add:

➢ Orange 5%

➢ Pineapple 5%

➢ Custard 5%

Let sit for three days at least; five days is best. Squeeze it a few time then shake each day for best results.

Sweet Mint Watermelon

Start with PG/VG/Nicotine based on your choice and add:

➢ Sweetener 10%

➢ Watermelon 5%

➢ Concentrated Menthol 1%

Tropical Lemonade

Start with PG/VG/Nicotine based on your choice and add:

➢ Strawberry 5%

- ➢ Peach 5%

- ➢ Coconut 3%

- ➢ Lemonade 5%

Sweet Tropical Fruit

Start with PG/VG/Nicotine based on your choice and add:

- ➢ Coconut 2%

- ➢ Pineapple 3%

- ➢ Strawberry 5%

- ➢ Watermelon 5%

Berry Cream

Start with PG/VG/Nicotine based on your choice and add:

- ➢ Blueberry 5%

- ➢ Strawberry 5%

- ➢ Cherry 2%

- ➢ Cream or Vanilla 2%

➢ Sweetener 1%

Give all flavors a hot water bath for at least an hour.

Tropical Cream

Start with PG/VG/Nicotine based on your choice and add:

➢ Watermelon 5%

➢ Peach 2%

➢ Strawberry 2%

➢ Pomegranate 1%

➢ Cream or Vanilla 1%

➢ Sweetener 1%

Chocolate/Caramel Orange

Start with PG/VG/Nicotine based on your choice and add:

➢ Chocolate 9%

➢ Orange 5%

➢ Caramel 1%

Sweet Fruit

Start with PG/VG/Nicotine based on your choice and add:

➤ Orange 3%

➤ Bubblegum 3%

➤ Black Cherry 3%

➤ Kiwi 3%

Sweet Pears

Start with PG/VG/Nicotine based on your choice and add:

➤ Pear 10%

➤ Coconut 3%

➤ Sweetener 2%

Strawberry Banana Ice Cream

Start with PG/VG/Nicotine based on your choice and add:

➤ Banana 5%

➤ Strawberry 5%

➢ Ice Cream 5%

Peaches and Cream

Start with PG/VG/Nicotine based on your choice and add:

➢ Peach 8%

➢ Cream or Vanilla 5%

➢ Pomegranate 3%

➢ Ethyl Maltol 1%

Steep for one week.

Melon Mint

Start with PG/VG/Nicotine based on your choice and add:

➢ Honey Dew Melon 10%

➢ Mint 5%

➢ Sweetener 2%

Steep for one week.

Lychee

Start with PG/VG/Nicotine based on your choice and add:

➤ Lychee 10%

➤ Cream or Vanilla 3%

➤ Sweetener 2%

Melon/Pear Dream

Start with PG/VG/Nicotine based on your choice and add:

➤ Melon 5%

➤ Pear 5%

Banana Fruit Cream

Start with PG/VG/Nicotine based on your choice and add:

➤ Orange 5%

➤ Cream or Vanilla 2%

➤ Banana 3%

➤ Strawberry 5%

Banana/Strawberry Custard Cream

Start with PG/VG/Nicotine based on your choice and add:

➢ Banana 5%

➢ Strawberry 5%

➢ Custard 3%

➢ Whipped Cream 2%

Peach Melon

Start with PG/VG/Nicotine based on your choice and add:

➢ Peach 5%

➢ Watermelon 3%

➢ Honeydew Melon 3%

Creamy Fruit Fritz

Start with PG/VG/Nicotine based on your choice and add:

➢ Watermelon 5%

➢ Kiwi 5%

- ➢ Peach 5%

- ➢ Cream or Vanilla 1%

- ➢ Ethyl maltol 1%

Peach Mint

Start with PG/VG/Nicotine based on your choice and add:

- ➢ Peach 10%

- ➢ Ethyl Maltol 1%

Steep a couple of days.

Minty Honeysuckle/Blueberry

Start with PG/VG/Nicotine based on your choice and add:

- ➢ Blueberry 5%

- ➢ Honeysuckle 5%

- ➢ Ethyl Maltol 3%

Banana Butterscotch

Start with PG/VG/Nicotine based on your choice and add:

➢ Butterscotch 5%

➢ Banana 10%

Minty Blueberry

Start with PG/VG/Nicotine based on your choice and add:

➢ Blueberry 14%

➢ Peppermint Oil 1%

Tropical Peach/Strawberry

Start with PG/VG/Nicotine based on your choice and add:

➢ Strawberry 5%

➢ Peach 5%

➢ Coconut 5%

Minty Apple

Start with PG/VG/Nicotine based on your choice and add:

➢ Green Apple 10%

➢ Ethyl Maltol 3%

Berry Cream Mint

Start with PG/VG/Nicotine based on your choice and add:

➢ Strawberry 5%

➢ Blueberry 5%

➢ Cream or Vanilla 5%

➢ Ethyl Maltol 4%

Watermelon Strawberry

Start with PG/VG/Nicotine based on your choice and add:

➢ Watermelon 5%

➢ Strawberry 5%

Banana Strawberry

Start with PG/VG/Nicotine based on your choice and add:

- ➢ Strawberry 5%

- ➢ Banana 5%

- ➢ Sweetener 3%

Banana Caramel Pudding

Start with PG/VG/Nicotine based on your choice and add:

- ➢ Caramel 5%

- ➢ Cream or Vanilla 5%

- ➢ Banana 4%

- ➢ MTS Vape Wizard 1%

Bakery / Dessert Recipes

Butterscotch Cookies

Start with PG/VG/Nicotine based on your choice and add:

- ➢ Butterscotch 5%

- ➢ Cream or Vanilla 5%

- ➢ Cookie 5%

➢ Sweetener 1%

Cinnamon Cake

Start with PG/VG/Nicotine based on your choice and add:

➢ Cake Batter 5%

➢ Cinnamon 2%

➢ Caramel 2%

➢ Sweetener 1%

You can vape immediately or steep for 24 hours.

Berry Muffin

Start with PG/VG/Nicotine based on your choice and add:

➢ Donut 5%

➢ Cream or Vanilla 1%

➢ Blueberry 5%

➢ Strawberry 4%

➢ Cinnamon 1%

Steep one to five days.

Sweet Key Lime Pie

Start with PG/VG/Nicotine based on your choice and add:

- ➢ Cheesecake 5%

- ➢ Graham Cracker 3%

- ➢ Cream or Vanilla 3%

- ➢ Key Lime 2%

Steep for a few days.

Peach/Apple Cobbler

Start with PG/VG/Nicotine based on your choice and add:

- ➢ Peach 5%

- ➢ Apple Pie 5%

Blueberry Cream

Start with PG/VG/Nicotine based on your choice and add:

- ➢ Blueberry 5%

- ➢ Vanilla 8%

- ➢ Cookie 2%

Steep 7 days.

Apple Cream

Start with PG/VG/Nicotine based on your choice and add:

- ➢ Cinnamon 2%

- ➢ Apple Pie 10%

- ➢ Cream or Vanilla 4%

Steep for five to seven days.

Sweet Strawberry Cheesecake

Start with PG/VG/Nicotine based on your choice and add:

- ➢ Strawberry 7%

- ➢ Cream or Vanilla 8%

- ➢ Cheesecake 3%

➢ Sweetener 1%

Honey Cream

Start with PG/VG/Nicotine based on your choice and add:

➢ Honey 5%

➢ Cream or Vanilla 10%

Hot Fudge Sunday

Start with PG/VG/Nicotine based on your choice and add:

➢ Milk Chocolate 5%

➢ Banana 5%

➢ Cherry 2%

➢ Cream or Vanilla 5%

➢ Whipped Cream 5%

Strawberry Cream Pie

Start with PG/VG/Nicotine based on your choice and add:

- ➤ Cream or Vanilla 5%

- ➤ Graham Cracker 2%

- ➤ Cheesecake 3%

- ➤ Strawberry 8%

- ➤ Custard 4%

- ➤ Ethyl Maltol 2%

Steep five days.

Dragon/Blueberry Cheesecake

Start with PG/VG/Nicotine based on your choice and add:

- ➤ Blueberry 5%

- ➤ Butter 3%

- ➤ Cheesecake 4%

- ➤ Dragon Fruit 5%

- ➤ Cream or Vanilla 2%

- ➤ Sweetener 2%

Steep for a few days.

Butterscotch Custard

Start with PG/VG/Nicotine based on your choice and add:

➢ Custard 10%

➢ Butterscotch 5%

➢ Whipped Cream 2%

Butterscotch/Banana/Rum Bread

Start with PG/VG/Nicotine based on your choice and add:

➢ Banana 5%

➢ Butterscotch 2%

➢ Caramel 2%

➢ Butter Rum 1%

➢ Brown Sugar 1%

Vape immediately or let steep a few days.

Sweet Yellow Cake

Start with PG/VG/Nicotine based on your choice and add:

- ➢ Yellow Cake 5%

- ➢ Vanilla or Cream 10%

- ➢ Sweetener 5%

Buttery Goodness

Start with PG/VG/Nicotine based on your choice and add:

- ➢ Butterscotch 5%

- ➢ Caramel 5%

- ➢ Cream or Vanilla 4%

- ➢ Cotton Candy 1%

Steep overnight.

Rice Crispy Treats

Start with PG/VG/Nicotine based on your choice and add:

- ➢ Marshmallow 5%

- ➢ Butter 5%

- ➢ Yellow Cake 5%

Peanut Butter Delight

Start with PG/VG/Nicotine based on your choice and add:

➢ Peanut Butter 5%

➢ Cookie 5%

➢ Vanilla 3%

➢ Sugar Cream 2%

Banana Cream Cookies

Start with PG/VG/Nicotine based on your choice and add:

➢ Banana 5%

➢ Cream or Vanilla 5%

➢ Sugar Cookie 5%

Creamy Cinnamon Roll

Start with PG/VG/Nicotine based on your choice and add:

➢ Cinnamon Roll 10%

➢ Cream or Vanilla 5%

Gingerbread Caramel Custard

Start with PG/VG/Nicotine based on your choice and add:

➢ Gingerbread 5%

➢ Custard 5%

➢ Caramel 4%

➢ Vanilla 1%

Candy Recipes

Hot Guava

Start with PG/VG/Nicotine based on your choice and add:

➢ Cotton Candy 8%

➢ Guava 3%

➢ Cinnamon 4%

Andes Mints

Start with PG/VG/Nicotine based on your choice and add:

➢ Chocolate 10%

- ➢ Crème De Menthe 3%

- ➢ Dulce De Leche 3%

- ➢ Sweetener 3%

Cantaloupe/Peach Rings with Cream

Start with PG/VG/Nicotine based on your choice and add:

- ➢ Peach 10%

- ➢ Cantaloupe 5%

- ➢ Cream or Vanilla 2%

Fruity Gum

Start with PG/VG/Nicotine based on your choice and add:

- ➢ Tutti Fruity 5%

- ➢ Bubble Gum 5%

- ➢ Cotton Candy 5%

Popcorn Treat

Start with PG/VG/Nicotine based on your choice and add:

- ➤ Popcorn 5%

- ➤ Caramel 5%

- ➤ Peanut Butter 5%

- ➤ Hazelnut 2%

- ➤ Cream or Vanilla 2%

Steep five days.

Caramel Vanilla

Start with PG/VG/Nicotine based on your choice and add:

- ➤ Caramel 10%

- ➤ Vanilla 5%

Mint Cream Butterscotch Toffee Caramel

Start with PG/VG/Nicotine based on your choice and add:

- ➤ Butterscotch 5%

- ➤ Caramel 4%

- ➢ Toffee 5%

- ➢ Cream or Vanilla 1%

- ➢ Ethyl Maltol 1%

Steep for seven days.

Minty Goodness

Start with PG/VG/Nicotine based on your choice and add:

- ➢ Peppermint 5%

- ➢ Spearmint 5%

Steep for one to two days.

Peanut Butter/Caramel Chocolate

Start with PG/VG/Nicotine based on your choice and add:

- ➢ Peanut Butter 5%

- ➢ Marshmallow 5%

- ➢ Chocolate 5%

- ➢ Caramel 3%

➢ Sweetener 1%

Steep for one week.

Coconut Chocolate

Start with PG/VG/Nicotine based on your choice and add:

➢ Chocolate 5%

➢ Coconut 5%

➢ Creme or Vanilla 5%

Yummy Drink Recipes

Irish Cream

Start with PG/VG/Nicotine based on your choice and add:

➢ Butterscotch 5%

➢ Irish Cream 5%

➢ Custard 3%

➢ Caramel 3%

➢ Cream or Vanilla 4%

Spicy Cinnamon

Start with PG/VG/Nicotine based on your choice and add:

➢ Cinnamon 3%

➢ Donut 5%

➢ Cereal 3%

➢ Sweetener 5%

Warm water bath and steep 2 days.

Energy Burn

Start with PG/VG/Nicotine based on your choice and add:

➢ Energy Drink 10%

➢ Cinnamon 5%

Hot Toddy

Start with PG/VG/Nicotine based on your choice and add:

➢ Brandy 5%

➢ Vanilla or Cream 5%

- ➢ Chocolate or Cocoa 5%

- ➢ Cinnamon 2%

Steep three days.

Tropical Rum

Start with PG/VG/Nicotine based on your choice and add:

- ➢ Orange 5%

- ➢ Mango 5%

- ➢ Rum 5%

Lemonade

Start with PG/VG/Nicotine based on your choice and add:

- ➢ Lemon 5%

- ➢ Orange 5%

- ➢ Kiwi Strawberry 5%

Steep two hours.

Exotic Tropics

Start with PG/VG/Nicotine based on your choice and add:

- ➤ Apricot 3%

- ➤ Guava 2%

- ➤ Mango 2%

- ➤ Passion Fruit 2%

- ➤ Orange 1%

Rose Cream

Start with PG/VG/Nicotine based on your choice and add:

- ➤ Rose 10%

- ➤ Cream or Vanilla 5%

Steep one to two weeks.

Creamy Cinnamon Chai Tea

Start with PG/VG/Nicotine based on your choice and add:

- ➤ Chai Tea 10%

- ➢ Cinnamon 1%

- ➢ Vanilla or Cream 3%

Sweet Tea with Lemon

Start with PG/VG/Nicotine based on your choice and add:

- ➢ Tea 10%

- ➢ Lemon 4%

- ➢ Sweetener 4%

- ➢ Menthol 1%

Cinnamon Chai Latte

Start with PG/VG/Nicotine based on your choice and add:

- ➢ Chai Tea 10%

- ➢ Cinnamon 1%

Tropical Vanilla Coke

Start with PG/VG/Nicotine based on your choice and add:

- ➢ Vanilla or Cream 10%

- ➢ Cola 2%

- ➢ Strawberry 2%

- ➢ Pineapple 1%

Tropical Orange Slurpee

Start with PG/VG/Nicotine based on your choice and add:

- ➢ Orange 10%

- ➢ Mango 5%

- ➢ Pineapple 2%

- ➢ Strawberry 2%

- ➢ Menthol 1%

Raspberry Lemonade

Start with PG/VG/Nicotine based on your choice and add:

- ➢ Lemonade 10%

- ➢ Raspberry 5%

Sweet Strawberry Lemonade

Start with PG/VG/Nicotine based on your choice and add:

➤ Strawberry 10%

➤ Lemon 5%

➤ Sweetener 2%

Caramel Coffee

Start with PG/VG/Nicotine based on your choice and add:

➤ Coffee 5%

➤ Praline and Cream 5%

➤ Caramel 4%

➤ Marshmallow 4%

Lemonade with Grape

Start with PG/VG/Nicotine based on your choice and add:

➤ Grape 10%

➤ Lemon 5%

Tropical Berry

Start with PG/VG/Nicotine based on your choice and add:

➢ Raspberry 5%

➢ Mango 3%

➢ Pineapple 5%

➢ Strawberry 5%

Tropical Coffee

Start with PG/VG/Nicotine based on your choice and add:

➢ Amaretto 5%

➢ Mango 5%

➢ Pineapple 5%

Milkshake with Strawberry

Start with PG/VG/Nicotine based on your choice and add:

➢ Strawberry 10%

➢ Cream or Vanilla 5%

Top 11 Recipes

Christmas

Start with PG/VG/Nicotine based on your choice and add:

- Cheesecake 3%

- Custard 4%

- Cream or Vanilla 3%

- Holiday Spice 2%

- Orange 1%

- Coconut 1%

- Peppermint 1%

Steep six days.

Creamy Berry Crunch

Start with PG/VG/Nicotine based on your choice and add:

- Strawberry 5%

- Cream or Vanilla 5%

- Cheesecake 5%

> ➢ Ethyl Maltol 1%

Hawaiian Pizza

Start with PG/VG/Nicotine based on your choice and add:

> ➢ Pizza 10%

> ➢ Pineapple 2%

> ➢ Bacon 2%

> ➢ Hickory Smoke 1%

Honeysuckle Cream

Start with PG/VG/Nicotine based on your choice and add:

> ➢ Honeysuckle 10%

> ➢ Vanilla 5%

Caramel/Toffee Cream

Start with PG/VG/Nicotine based on your choice and add:

> ➢ Caramel 5%

- ➢ Cream or Vanilla 5%

- ➢ Toffee 5%

Toffee/Caramel Cookie

Start with PG/VG/Nicotine based on your choice and add:

- ➢ Toffee 5%

- ➢ Caramel 5%

- ➢ White Chocolate 2%

- ➢ Cookie 2%

Cappuccino

Start with PG/VG/Nicotine based on your choice and add:

- ➢ Cappuccino 4%

- ➢ Toffee 4%

- ➢ Whipped Cream 4%

- ➢ Caramel 4%

Berry Caramel Cream

Start with PG/VG/Nicotine based on your choice and add:

➢ Cream or Vanilla 15%

➢ Caramel 1%

➢ Cheesecake 5%

➢ Cinnamon 1%

➢ Graham Cracker 1%

➢ Marshmallow 1%

➢ Strawberry 5%

➢ Custard 2%

Strawberry Custard

Start with PG/VG/Nicotine based on your choice and add:

➢ Cream or Vanilla 5%

➢ Graham Crust 1%

➢ Cheesecake 2%

➢ Strawberry 5%

- ➢ Custard 2%

Steep three to fourteen days.

Tropical Coconut

Start with PG/VG/Nicotine based on your choice and add:

- ➢ Pear 5%

- ➢ Peach 5%

- ➢ Coconut 1%

- ➢ Donuts 2%

Saltwater Taffy

Start with PG/VG/Nicotine based on your choice and add:

- ➢ Saltwater Taffy 10%

- ➢ Blueberry 5%

- ➢ Grape 3%

- ➢ Smooth 2%

- ➢ Cream or Vanilla 2%

> Sweetener 1%

Pineapple/Coconut Cream

Start with PG/VG/Nicotine based on your choice and add:

> Pineapple 5%

> Coconut 5%

> Cream or Vanilla 5%

Steep for a week.

Berry Mint Cream

Start with PG/VG/Nicotine based on your choice and add:

> Strawberry 5%

> Blueberry 5%

> Cream or Vanilla 5%

> Dolce De Lechee 2%

> Sweetener 1%

> Ethyl Maltol 1%

Tropical Mojito

Start with PG/VG/Nicotine based on your choice and add:

➢ Papaya 3%

➢ Lychee 2%

➢ Key Lime 3%

➢ Mango 4%

➢ Jackfruit 5%

➢ Menthol 1%

Creamy Blueberry/Pomegranate

Start with PG/VG/Nicotine based on your choice and add:

➢ Vanilla 4%

➢ Blueberry 5%

➢ Pomegranate 3%

Cinnamon Sugar Cookie

Start with PG/VG/Nicotine based on your choice and add:

➢ Cinnamon 5%

- ➢ Cinnamon Sugar Cookie 10%

- ➢ Vanilla or Cream 4%

- ➢ Toasted Almond 1%

Mint Delight

Start with PG/VG/Nicotine based on your choice and add:

- ➢ Cream de Menthe 3%

- ➢ Menthol 5%

- ➢ Sweetener 2%

- ➢ Peppermint 5%

Coconut/Pear Cream

Start with PG/VG/Nicotine based on your choice and add:

- ➢ Pear 5%

- ➢ Cream or Vanilla 3%

- ➢ Coconut 2%

E-Juice Vendors

NOW THAT we've looked at the basics of making your own flavors and given you some good recipe options to start with, where can you go for trustworthy and organic e-juice flavors? I'm going to tell you of the two best e-juice organic vendors.

VirginVapor.com

This is one of the biggest organic e-juice vendors on the market today. Based in California, this company is one of the true organic manufacturers in the US, and their mission statement says they rely on the fact that organic tastes better.

None of the e-liquids from this company contain artificial flavorings, colors, sweeteners or other additives. They are also vegan, GMO-free and contain no gluten or sugar. Their basic ingredients are the following:

✧ Pharmaceutical grade Kosher nicotine

✧ Organic pharmaceutical grade vegetable glycerin

✧ Pure, distilled water

✧ Certified organic flavors

All e-liquid from Virgin Vapor are tested to be free of DEG, mercury, lead, chromium and cadmium. All of their flavors come in glass bottles, not plastic, to avoid chemicals such as BPA from leaching into the e-liquid.

Virgin Vapor features e-liquid that is 100% VG based. Most e-juice are advertised as VG based, but still, contain PG; but not at Virgin Vapor. However, they thin their VG bases juices with pure, distilled water to get the thinness of PG. Lastly, the nicotine in Virgin Vapor products is 100% USA made from tobacco leaves grown in North Carolina.

Kind Juice

This Florida-based business is on the short list of pure e-juice vendors. They offer complex flavor tones, with careful attention to natural and raw ingredients. In order to be an organic e-juice, it needs to be 100% VG. Kind Juice does this by using only natural VG, produced from plants grown without pesticides and extracted through a natural process.

Kind Juice also sources all of their nicotine from USA tobacco crops that are ethically grown without pesticides or growth control agents, striving to keep results as pure as possible. They use no chemicals or solvents in a cold/closed refinement process to shield the nicotine from light, heat and oxygen to give you a pure nicotine with a smoother and cleaner flavor. This also gives the juice an extended shelf-life.

Natures Flavors.com

This online retailer sells organic food grade flavor extracts. I tried their strawberry flavor, and I liked it, it was not the very best (the best was a non-organic one), but hey we are talking organic right?

BareNakedJuice.com

Once again please understand I am not endorsing any of these companies, nor will I get any affiliate commission from them, so my advice is, do your own research and see what you can find. I just bought some flavors from each of them and as I said I have had better, but those mostly were non-organic.

Have you ever tried a candy call Laffy Taffy, if so Banana flavored ones, or have you ever tried a candy call the Fireball? See when you try either of them, you will think wow what a beautiful flavor of banana or this is really sweet and spicy cinnamon right? But in actuality, a real banana or actual cinnamon do not taste that good. My point is just because it is organic doesn't mean it will taste 100 times better, no, but hey you will at least be smoking something that has fewer harmful chemical. So be happy.

Last Word

I HAVE MENTIONED over 35 flavors in these recipes. If you are about to try and make a few bottles for yourself, one word of advice, please don't go buy 15-20 of these flavors at first. Instead, buy 2-3 max, start off easy start slow and see if you like the taste if you like the experience of making your own e-liquid first. Then once you know, you enjoy the process, and you love the taste of your own creation, buy more flavors.

As I said before, when it comes to organic flavors, often you can extract the flavor from a fruit or herb (vanilla) and make the juice yourself, but I highly urge you not to try that. I have tried it, and it never turns out good.

Instead, pick an online or local retailers who carry organic flavor extracts and buy from them. At first, you may have to buy one bottle from each vendor and see whose taste the best then start buying from them. Just because I said I love John Doe Company's banana flavor doesn't mean when you try it, you will feel the same way about it. We all have very unique and individual taste buds, so what maybe awesome to me will not be the same for you.

My writing skills are not the best, but the information I provide is 100% authentic, that much I can assure you. Vaping is a passion of mine and it has been for many years now.

If you think I have provided you with quality information, I would love to see a book review from you, it would mean a lot to me honestly.

If you would like to get in touch with me, please feel free to email me at: evapelite@gmail.com

Thank you once again for buying my book.

Happy Vaping friends!

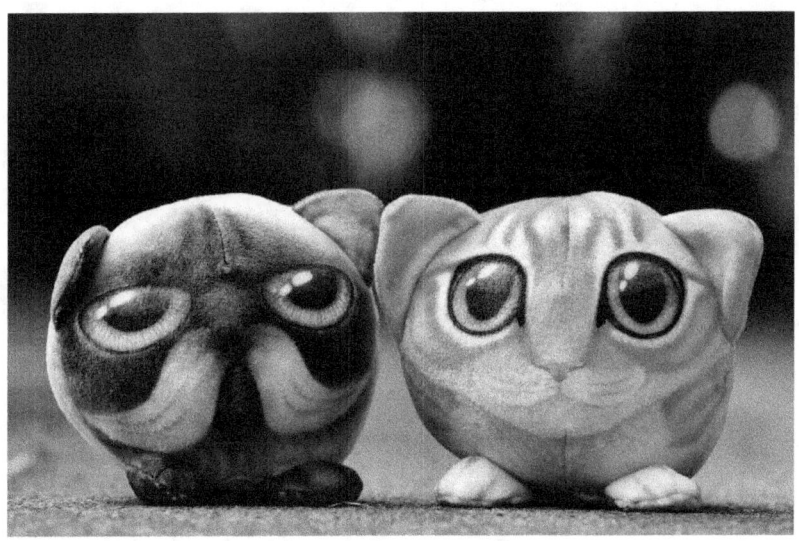

www.ingramcontent.com/pod-product-compliance
Lightning Source LLC
Chambersburg PA
CBHW060207290526
45789CB00003B/1192

* 9 7 8 1 5 4 1 2 5 5 5 2 4 *